Optimize Your Healthcare Supply Chain Performance: A Strategic Approach

This book is dedicated to God as well as to our families, mentors, friends, and colleagues, who sustain us and enrich our lives. Thank you for supporting us with love, advice, collaborative energy, and friendship.

Your board, staff, or clients may also benefit from this book's insight. For more information on quantity discounts, contact the Health Administration Press Marketing Manager at (312) 424-9470.

Library of Congress Cataloging-in-Publication Data

Ledlow, Gerald R.
    Optimize your healthcare supply chain performance : a strategic approach / Gerald R. Ledlow, Allison P. Corry, Mark A. Cwiek.
        p. cm.
    Includes Bibliographical referances (p).
    ISBN-13: 978-1-56793-950-7 (alk. paper)
    ISBN-10: 1-56793-950-3(alk. paper)
    1. Health facilities—Materials management. 2. Business logistics. 3. Medical supplies. I. Corry, Allison. II. Cwiek, Mark A. III. Title.
    RA971.33.L43 2007
    362.1068'7—dc22

                                                                    2006046998

The paper used in this publication meets the minimum requirements of American National Standard for Information Sciences—Permanence of Paper for Printed Library Materials, ANSI Z39.48-1984. ∞ ™

Acquisitions editor: Audrey Kaufman; Project manager: Amanda Bove; Layout editor: Chris Underdown; Cover designer: Betsy Pérez

Health Administration Press
A division of the Foundation of the
    American College of Healthcare Executives
1 North Franklin Street, Suite 1700
Chicago, IL 60606-3529
(312) 424-2800

Introduction

As for the future, your task is not to foresee it, but to enable it.

—Antoine de Saint-Exupéry

This book was written with the busy healthcare executive in mind. Its purpose is to provide senior healthcare executives and other key leaders with an understanding of different supply chain structures and effective management tenets for those structures. Strategies are presented in this book with the goal of optimizing high-level decision making that is focused on developing a solid foundation for supply chain operations and management. By the end of this book, the reader will have a good grasp of important executive-level trade-offs, benefits, costs, and options within supply chain operations and management. ▸

The stakes in healthcare have never been higher. Gone are the relatively forgiving days of cost reimbursement and loose pricing accountabilities. The degree to which discounting, managed care, and regulation have pushed the risks and consequences of supply chain inefficiencies upon the provider could not have been imagined a decade ago. All providers are affected, including hospitals, healthcare systems, doctors, and medical clinics.

The financial environment can indeed be harsh within healthcare. On the other hand, healthcare leaders who inspire their teams to develop sound supply chain strategies can reap huge rewards. These rewards relate directly to clinical success, financial gain, and organizational morale.

In all industries, not just healthcare, three out of four chief executive officers (CEOs) consider their supply chains to be essential to gaining competitive advantage within their markets (Poirer and Quinn 2003). The most profitable organizations, often the acknowledged best companies in the world, have mastered the science and art of supply chain management. These organizations realized long ago that supply chain

management and improvement require total team commitment and effort. Healthcare organizations, individually and as an industry, have been a decade or more behind other industries in understanding effective supply chain structure, coordination, management, and value.

Today's healthcare leaders are well aware of the mounting pressures to provide documented, positive outcomes of patient care and to reduce costs whenever possible while providing that care. Healthcare leaders have learned to operate in the environment of shrinking and often negative margins. It only makes sense that healthcare leaders are seizing the opportunity to rise to a higher mastery of supply chain management and oversight. This book seeks to provide an overview of two very different healthcare supply chain models, to present strategic factors important to improving supply chain management, and to discuss supply chain value principles.

The information in this book will help healthcare leaders make important and reasonable decisions to improve the organization's supply chain system. Selecting where to make changes, when to use different approaches, and how to find greater value are at the very heart of this book. The decisions and implementation processes can be incremental (an adaptive change model) or dramatic (such as in the "best practice" approach). The main lesson to be learned is that improving the supply chain system begins where one is today, and that the organization can strive to continuously improve and optimize the system over time. One thing is certain: There is sufficient evidence to indicate that healthcare leaders need to attend to their supply chain at a much greater level than in the past.

Supply chain improvement can be fulfilling as a multiprofessional team endeavor, exciting as a monitored set of achievable goals, and rewarding as a key part of financial success. The authors wish you fulfilling, exciting, and rewarding times ahead.

REFERENCES

Poirer, C., and F. Quinn. 2003. "A Survey of Supply Chain Progress." *Supply Chain Management Review* (Sept./Oct.). [Online article; retrieved 4/21/06.] http://www.manufacturing.net/scm/article/CA323602.html?text = survey + of + supply + chain.

CHAPTER 1

Approaches to
Healthcare Supply Chain

Good plans shape good decisions. That's why good planning helps to make elusive dreams come true.

—*Lester R. Bittel,* The Nine Master Keys of Management

This chapter describes several major issues in supply chain management that have been identified by senior healthcare leaders and experts. The range of options that an organization's supply chain management system can adopt in response to the issues it faces is represented as a spectrum. On one end of the spectrum is the most common approach, the traditional model, which is highly dependent on outside intermediaries, such as group purchasing organizations (GPOs), distribution organizations, and transportation organizations. On the other end of the spectrum is the vertically integrated model, which is structured to be less dependent on outside intermediaries and more controlled by the healthcare organization, and thus it can be viewed as a more "dis-intermediated" model. In between, there is a range of structure possibilities available to healthcare leadership. ▶

There are many possible hybrid, or "in between," models of supply chain structures. For example, the medical and surgical supply items in a supply chain may use a vertically integrated model approach, while the pharmaceutical items may use the traditional model structure. Also, service lines or service-line components, such as cardiac rhythm management, may use the vertically integrated model approach, while the majority of the supply chain operation embraces the traditional model. To understand what structure or model to use, leaders must determine what approach to use for the supply chain; each supply chain component can be structured to the advantage of the organization.

Healthcare organizations should develop a new vision for supply chain management that is coupled with an appreciation and understanding of the continuum represented by these two models. With that understanding, the organization will be better equipped to move deliberately toward the realm of systemwide and purposeful internal control— the vertically integrated side of the spectrum. At a minimum, healthcare organizations should be better prepared to more effectively manage the traditional model elements of its system.

MAJOR ISSUES FROM THE CEO'S PERSPECTIVE

How can the leader in a health organization best ensure improved, and even optimal, supply chain performance? What facilitating factors and principles are vital for creating a strategic foundation to effectively and efficiently deliver care, taking into account the need for interaction within the greater supply chain? This book addresses the above two questions and illustrates the imperatives of the healthcare supply chain with regard to structure, pricing, volume, utilization, and technology.

In e-mail correspondence on February 15, 2006, author Dr. Gerald Ledlow asked experts within healthcare supply chain operations about the major issues that CEOs need to address with regard to supply chain management. Among the respondents were Terry Cox of HCA in Nashville, Tennessee, and Vance Moore and Marita Parks of Sisters of Mercy Health Systems in Saint Louis, Missouri. Clearly, there needs to be an effort to encourage providers to take ownership of their supply chain as a strategic and essential part of the provision of care. A summary of their insights highlights the need to create systematic approaches to

- Reduce ambiguities and align accountabilities among those who sell, make product decisions, pay, and reimburse while linking product selection to clinical outcomes so that the real value of product choices can be objectively evaluated;
- Keep up with the rapid proliferation of technology and supplies with a bias toward value;
- Attract and keep professional supply chain experts within an industry that does not fully appreciate the essential role that supply chain can play;
- Manage pharmaceuticals and physician preference items, particularly in cardiology and orthopedic service lines;
- Find and realize supply chain operational savings, such as maintaining stock keeping unit (SKU) standardization and developing compression to fewer, more widely used supply items; and

- Improve leadership and team understanding with regard to how to maximize the value of leverage through properly managed purchase volume.

Systems require a foundation comprised of a solid base of knowledge and an effective infrastructure to be successful. As in all systems, the effectiveness of one area affects the effectiveness of other areas. Indeed, the healthcare supply chain impacts patient care delivery, satisfaction levels of all stakeholders, and the financial health of an organization.

While financial impact is very important, there are additional considerations, including patient safety, physician and nurse satisfaction, and improved patient care and patient satisfaction (NPSF 2000). Consider for a moment the impact of "stock-outs," pilfered items, damaged items, and misplaced items on the delivery of patient care. In many healthcare organizations, improving the supply chain has yielded concomitant improvements to patient safety and clinician satisfaction.

To understand the healthcare supply chain, it is important to be able to recognize traits of the traditional model (also known as the "intermediated model" because of its dependency on the intermediaries in the chain) on one end of the spectrum and the traits of the more contemporary model on the other end, the vertically integrated model, which is limited in its intermediary involvement. Figure 1.1 shows the different levels of intermediary involvement in the two models. Of course, a healthcare organization may operate at any point along the spectrum; this chapter will explore the relative benefits and trade-offs of various placements within the spectrum.

TRADITIONAL MODEL

Today's healthcare supply chain follows the traditional model. Supply chain management in the United States needs a new vision, but to imagine a better future, one must first know what can be improved. It would be helpful to consider the following list of characteristics of today's healthcare supply chain (the traditional model) and relate them to your own supply chain:

■ *Multiple systems with multiple processes that lack cohesiveness*

Figure 1.1. Intermediary Involvement Across the Supply Chain Spectrum

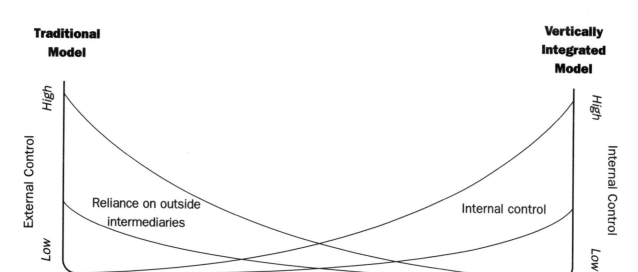

and uniformity. Many health systems and stand-alone facilities use different materials management information systems and different processes across facilities and departments.

- *High distributor fees.* Most healthcare organizations spend hundreds of thousands of dollars or more on outside parties for supply (mainly medical/surgical and pharmaceutical) distribution.

- *Service quality failures and service frequency do not match need.* Distributors commonly fill only 80 percent to 90 percent of the order. This causes a large number of product shortages for clinicians each day, which is a service quality failure. At other times, distributors overfill orders, causing excessive stock on shelves and higher costs for the overage and for storage. As for frequency, many healthcare organizations receive supplies based on distributors' schedules rather than clinical needs.

- *Wholesalers lead pharmacy processes.* The outside distributors/wholesalers who supply the medications control the systems and processes for medication sourcing, ordering, receiving, and distribution.

- *Inconsistent management processes.* It is not unusual for a facility to have different departments that manage the supply chain in different ways. They may have separate information systems, different inventory systems, and even different basic nomenclature.

- *Limited usable data.* In many healthcare organizations, identical products have different names depending on the facility and/or department. This limits an organization's ability to aggregate data for decision making, volume purchasing, and bulk ordering (thus affecting the bottom line) and presents a potential communication barrier between materials management and clinical end users.

- *Many intermediaries.* The majority of distributors service many customers and stock what sells best for them (not necessarily what the provider needs or wants). This means that healthcare organizations get supplies from many different distribution facilities to meet their needs or are directed to use what the distributor stocks in that particular service region.

Most healthcare organizations live in the world just described. This puts materials managers in the position of maintaining a supply chain of "weak links." Senior leaders reading this book need to reflect on the situation just described and envision a better way to operate the supply chain in their organizations.

The traditional model's structure and cost breakdown are illustrated in Figures 1.2 and 1.3, respectively. Figure 1.2 illustrates the heavy use of intermediaries in the traditional model. Figure 1.3 portrays total delivered costs—that is, the breakdown of costs to get a supply item from the manufacturer to the patient's bedside. The blocks in the first column, Manufacturer Company A, represent the portion of total delivered costs associated with the manufacturer's costs (e.g., for production, raw materials, machinery, plastics, and packaging) and the manufacturer's profit. The block in the second column, GPO Company B, represents the GPO's administrative costs for initiating, negotiating, maintaining, and marketing their group contracts with manufacturers and distributors. The blocks in the third and fourth

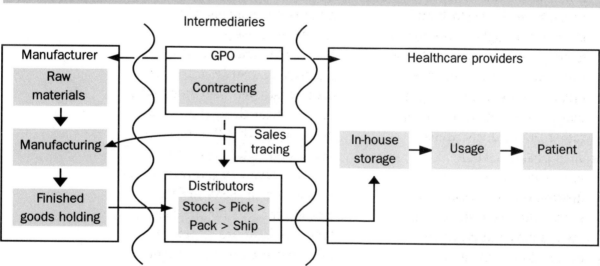

Figure 1.2. Traditional/Nonintegrated Healthcare Supply Chain Model Structure

Source: Adopted from McCurry et al. 2005.

Figure 1.3. Traditional Model Healthcare Supply Chain Costs

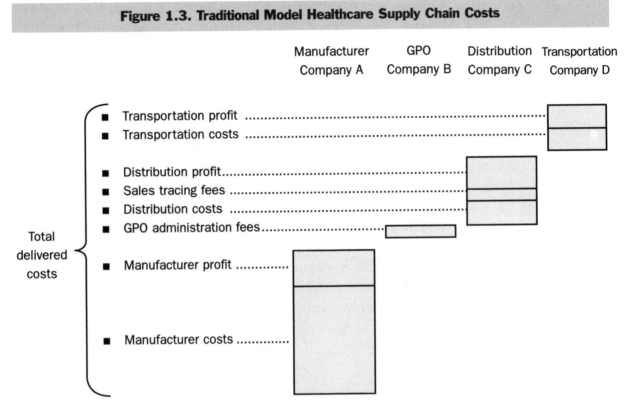

Source: Adopted from McCurry et al. 2005.

columns represent the portion of total delivered costs associated with the costs and profits of the distribution and transportation companies, respectively.

Conflicts

The traditional model creates an environment in which multiple entities, each involved to some degree with group purchasing, distribution, or transportation, add to the costs and reduce profits. This is not necessarily a negative aspect of the model if the hospital or health system receives a quality supply item, quality service, and a better price (thus lower cost) than what it could achieve by itself. However, not only are additional costs added to the system because of the various intermediaries involved in this model, but it is also difficult to align incentives to reduce supply chain items and operational costs.

Without aligned incentives, the various separate intermediaries may conflict with each other based on dollar flow and processes that maximize their profit margins. This is how the free marketplace works: The intermediaries are not "bad" but are merely attempting to maximize their profits. However, it is vital to understand that misaligned incentives have the greatest opportunity to exist in this model. Improvement opportunities for this model may be achieved by aligning incentives among the various entities, but this is difficult and time consuming.

Decision Points

The traditional model's stakeholders clearly have different incentives and goals within the overall healthcare supply chain. Understanding the structure, cost allocation, and incentives within the traditional model is key to making wise decisions about outsourcing or insourcing; the structure of the particular hospital or health system supply chain; and where to select different approaches to optimizing supply chain operations to achieve reduced costs, greater patient, physician, and clinical staff

satisfaction, and overall improved patient care. Swedish Health Services, as described in the following section, has improved upon the traditional supply chain model by aggressively taking control of internal processes, setting goals, and structuring intermediary influence on supply chain operations.

Case in Point: Swedish Health Services

Swedish Health Services, a not-for-profit system, has nearly 1,300 beds within four acute care facilities and staffs 7,000 employees and 1,500 physicians. Annually, over 40,000 procedures are performed for net revenues of $1.1 billion, and $170 million is spent on the supply chain. Using the traditional supply chain approach, Swedish realized that opportunities to positively affect its bottom line were being squandered. The health system looked to improve its traditional model, utilizing the "use our minds before we spend our bucks" philosophy. Highlights of the improvements at Swedish included the following (Caudle 2006):

■ A self-contracting model was developed that reduced the dependence on a GPO. Today, 94 percent of purchases are by contract.

- Attention and effort were focused on the item master and charge master data files to achieve a clean database and clear links across data tables. This means analyses and management will be based on good information.
- An intense vendor management program was adopted and implemented. Today, all vendors must wear an identification badge in all facilities, and a thorough testing and an evaluation of vendor compliance (service and quality) with system policies are conducted. This structures external entities'/vendors' interactions with the health system; health system team members are trained to only interact and work with properly credentialed and badged vendors.
- Better management of critical use equipment was achieved, especially for intravenous (IV) pumps, patient-controlled anesthesia pumps, and other like items. Goals were set and measured for critical equipment to include "up time" (the time before the equipment is ready to use), location of equipment, and associated supply item availability.

- Anesthesia and perioperative product management programs were developed and implemented.
- Intense supply chain management of the cardiac catheterization laboratory and interventional radiology service was implemented.

These efforts resulted in significant improvements. Supply chain spending, as a percentage of net revenue, dropped from 21 percent to 16.5 percent from 1999 to 2005 and saved $30 million from the operating expense in the bottom line (Caudle 2006). Swedish has achieved better control with improved quality of service, while at the same time reducing costs. Other improvements from this effort resulted in the following:

- Availability of critical use equipment increased to 99 percent, while costs were reduced from $12 to less than $1 per turn of the equipment.
- Because patient care staff were relieved of some supply chain tasks, they gained 15 minutes per shift to spend on patient care tasks. Inefficiencies were reduced in the supply chain so that clinical

staff could reduce the number of supply chain tasks that they had historically accomplished.

- Operating room turnover time was reduced from nearly 60 minutes to 34 minutes (using hospitality industry knowledge) because of enhanced supply chain efficiency in the reduced operating room case-cart preparation and improved housekeeping efficiency.
- Out-of-date medications in anesthesia were decreased from 30 percent to 1 percent.
- The number of times an operating room technician needs a supply item outside the operating room during a case decreased from eight to less than one because of improved case-cart preparation and the availability of high-use supply items in the operating room.
- Giving clinical staff in the cardiac catheterization laboratory more time for patient care tasks resulted in higher patient volume and turnover, as well as reduced supply items costs. The result was a 208 percent return on investment.
- Better overall contract terms and service and payment terms were achieved.

Swedish Health Services improved on the traditional model by using good business practices. It took some components of the vertically integrated model and used them where they would prove most valuable and advantageous. This is most apparent in the control of operating room and cardiac catheterization service-line supply items and processes and in the external entity/vendor-structured system for interaction with the health system. It structured external organization interaction with its health system, set internal goals, and measured and managed specific services lines that were most costly in the supply chain. The decision whether to outsource components of the traditional model is situational, and the evaluation of one's own particular business case can lead to great improvements.

VERTICALLY INTEGRATED MODEL

Healthcare supply chain management needs a better way to do business and to serve patients more effectively and efficiently. The existing traditional model supply chain needs to be strategically evaluated, leveraged, and used as a competitive advantage within the marketplace. The vertically integrated model incorporates these changes. Characteristics of this model are as follows.

Single System, Common Data, and Electronic Purchasing

An information system for materials management that is linked to finance (cost accounting and revenue) and clinical systems in a seamless environment using common data across the organization is vital for improving decision-support information and implementing projects aimed at cost savings and quality improvement. This also enables uniform analyses and consistent processes across the enterprise.

Considering that a manually processed order takes 40 percent of a purchaser/buyer's time and 68 percent of an account payables clerk's time and is seven times more expensive than an electronic order (Conway 2006), it is essential that purchasing move to an electronic system. The reduction of rework is evident in a single electronic system. The average cost of correcting single order discrepancies (cost shared between hospitals and suppliers) ranges from $15 to $50 each, and inconsistencies in ordering occur 35 percent of the time between health system/hospital supply data and supplier data (Conway 2006). If a hospital places 100 orders a week (most place many more), the annual cost of manual system discrepancies ranges from $27,300 to $91,000.

Over a decade ago, the following statement was published by *Medical Device & Diagnostic Industry* magazine:

In the United States, the Health Industry Distributors Association (HIDA) estimates that medical supplies and equipment account for $28 billion in healthcare costs annually. According to the Association, a significant portion of that healthcare bill could be trimmed through better communications. Workable standards for implementing a broadly based electronic data system already exist, and the accompanying technologies have been tested and refined over a decade in the retail and food industries" (Freiherr 1996).

A treasure trove of untapped opportunities still exist, ten years later, to use electronic communications to reduce costs.

Distributor Fee Reduction and/or Elimination

It is possible to reduce and in some cases eliminate the need for the middle links in the supply chain by working directly with distributors and manufacturers and by directly negotiating fees, shipment locations, and so forth. (Note that the opportunities to eliminate fees are also available in the traditional model by requiring distributors to bid for your business, which can initially reduce fees by up to 40 percent.)

Service and Quality Failure Reduction

Healthcare organizations can better control their supply chain service quality by negotiating with manufacturers and distributors. Considering supply and pharmaceutical items, it is important to firmly establish when, where, and within what ranges are acceptable service quality (for undersupply and oversupply fulfillment). Being specific on expectations and evaluating performance are critical to improving service and quality. The key measure is "service fulfillment rate"—simply,

did the undamaged item get delivered to the right place, at the right time, and in the correct quantity? Data from a single source and a seamless information system can also identify the items to stock internally, and in what quantities, for rapid response to clinicians. One health system, Sisters of Mercy Health System in Saint Louis, Missouri, made significant improvements in this area by eliminating over 3,000 product stock-outs (items needed but not available) each day across a 19-hospital system. This also yielded major gains in patient safety and clinician satisfaction. More information about the Sisters of Mercy's accomplishments are outlined later in this chapter.

Consistent Management Processes and Reduced Complexity

The ability to streamline and adopt consistent processes for ordering, purchasing, receiving, managing inventory, replenishing, and capturing charges for billable supply items is directly associated with improved bottom-line performance, patient safety, and stakeholder satisfaction. Consistent processes can be realized by dusting off the old standard operating procedures and making them usable, relevant documents. Process consistency is attained by training people on the established standard processes, insisting on compliance to the processes, rewarding compliance, and monitoring consistency. Many healthcare systems and hospitals have extended this concept by developing and operating a centralized supply-chain customer-service function and by centralizing, at least to some degree, the purchasing function. This effort, once implemented, greatly reduces the complexity of the supply chain as well, which leads to greater supply chain understanding and proficiency across the organization.

Reliable, When-Needed Service

Healthcare organizations that negotiate service delivery parameters with distributors are more likely to get supplies when and where they need them, even to every facility every day, than if they depend on distributor's service routes. This negotiation should be done in conjunction with distributor fees (fees distributors charge you for delivery).

Stocking What Is Needed

Single information systems, common data, and effective negotiation with distributors and manufacturers enable the healthcare organization to stock that which is really needed at that site and to no longer be dependent on what sells best for distributors. For example, items that have a history of "stock-outs" can be stocked internally and managed to improve patient safety and stakeholder satisfaction.

Benefits

The vertically integrated model uses insourcing to a much greater extent than the traditional model does. This model maintains an internal group purchasing, distribution, transportation, and hospital supply chain organization in which the goals and work are coordinated to derive the greatest value for the organization. Figures 1.4 and 1.5 depict the vertically integrated model's structure and cost and revenue allocation. As compared to the traditional model shown in Figure 1.2, the vertically integrated model focuses on direct connection to manufacturers, eliminates intermediaries (and their associated costs) as much as possible, and adds revenue to the healthcare

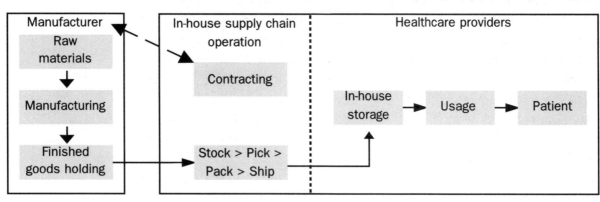

Figure 1.4. The Vertically Integrated Healthcare Supply Chain Model Structure

Source: Adopted from McCurry et al. 2005.

organization in the form of sales tracing and utilization reports (which are used to pay commissions to sales representatives and add information to manufacturer decision support systems regarding market penetration rates by region, organization, department, and in some cases by physician or surgeon).

In contrast to the traditional model, the vertically integrated model accomplishes the following:

- Eliminating external nonessential supply chain entities (GPOs and distributors)
- Insourcing the traditional model to speed transition and capture traditional revenue streams

- Increasing control and accountability for service, pricing, and quality
- Establishing closer links to manufacturers

The vertically integrated model can achieve a net savings on supply costs of 15 percent to 20 percent and can introduce a revenue stream from sales tracing reports of 1 percent to 5 percent, depending on the manufacturer. Of course, the larger the operation, the greater the economies of scope and scale that would compete with the traditional model costs of outsourcing. Also, the ability to positively improve patient safety and physician and staff satisfaction is enhanced by improving service

Figure 1.5. Cost and Revenue Comparison Between the Vertically Integrated Model and the Traditional Model

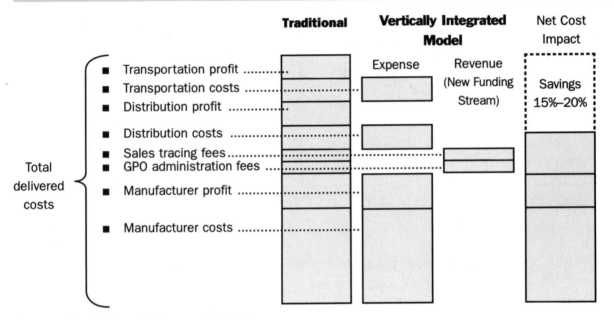

Source: Adopted from McCurry et al. 2005.

(timeliness and accuracy) and leveraging opportunities of compliance. Opportunities of compliance revolve around selecting one or two manufacturer service lines that represent high-priced and high-volume items, such as cardiac rhythm management supplies and implants, and leveraging better pricing due to volume and compliance. This also improves patient safety (a surgeon who implants the same brand of item 100 times should be better than one who implants five different brands, 20 times each), as well as clinician satisfaction when they are decisive factors in the decision process.

The vertically integrated model requires the healthcare organization to develop and build infrastructure to operate and supply resources to the supply chain. This includes creating and operating (1) an internal GPO or purchasing operation (consult federal regulations for legal status requirements, such as for-profit status and external customers); (2) a distribution system with warehousing capabilities, such as a consolidated services center; and (3) a transportation fleet over and above the typical in-house localized supply chain operation that is common in most hospitals. With the addition of the new structure, which replaces intermediary structures and processes, the healthcare organization is in a much better position to control all aspects of the supply chain.

Conflicts

Several conflicts can emerge from the vertically integrated model, both external and internal.

EXTERNAL. The healthcare industry likes tradition and doing things the way they were done in the past. The vertically integrated model is a departure from traditional supply chain forms. In the external battle, manufacturers, distributors, and transporters will attempt to ignore the vertically integrated model and will not recognize it for what it is. Examples of this are refusal to pay for sales tracing reports, slow receipt of contractual group discounts, and refusal to transport supply items directly to the healthcare organization (versus using a distributor). This means that they

will fight any attempt to steer funds from their profits. Therefore, perhaps the largest hurdle will be to win an external battle for recognition as a vertically integrated model in which compliance rebates and sales tracing fees are paid to the healthcare organization rather than to others. Recommendations for evaluating and working with external organizations are presented in Chapter 3.

Another conflict is in contracting and purchasing as a GPO or purchasing department. Contracting and negotiating under this model will steer funds to the healthcare organization, and other entities will try to thwart this approach. It is important to remember, in any event, that the healthcare organization has the ability to comply with contract terms (percent usage of an item under contract), where stand-alone, non-patient care delivery GPOs do not have that ability.

INTERNAL. There are internal conflicts as well, and most revolve around capital funding. During times of tighter resources, it may be politically impossible to move to a large-scale vertically integrated model. Certain components of the supply chain could move in that direction, however, creating a hybrid model that takes elements of both models and uses those elements to the greatest value for the organization. Conflicts can exist with physicians and clinical staff over supply item compression (reducing suppliers to get a discount price for items rather than working with many suppliers), selection, and compliance. Incentives therefore become important; for example, a percentage of bottom-line savings being returned or reinvested to the complying service line, or otherwise demonstrating the tangible monetary cost benefits associated with the utilization of contracted items.

Continually improving the services being provided internally and remaining competitive with externally based technology and service advancements are challenges that must be overcome with the constant reevaluation and improvement of the internally managed supply chain. With a creative team having mutually aligned incentives within the organization, those most familiar with the processes and corporate culture will push the envelope with value-added changes to improve the supply chain. These internal resources will be the developers of the organization's continuous improvement initiatives as the supply chain system matures.

Decision Points

There are several decision points in deciding if a vertically integrated model or some of its components is right for your healthcare organization. First consider whether capital funds can be dedicated to establish the infrastructure that is needed to create (1) a group purchasing capability; (2) a warehousing and inventory management capability, either inside or outside the facility; (3) a distribution system; and (4) an internal facility management capability. The second consideration is quantifying the anticipated benefit from the transition to an internally managed vertical supply chain management model. Some questions to ask include the following: What is the value of an overall system of control? What are the political incentives that need to be aligned in this model? What components of the vertically integrated supply chain will be most valuable for the scope and scale of operations? The strategic factor assessment tool provided in the next chapter can help with an initial evaluation of your healthcare organization.

Case in Point: Sisters of Mercy Health System

The Sisters of Mercy Health System embarked on a journey from 2002 through 2006 to change the traditional healthcare supply chain model to reap financial, patient safety, and clinician satisfaction benefits. From this effort, the current return on investment from the vertically integrated strategy is a $6 return per $1 invested in the operation. Figure 1.6 explains the evolution of this strategy.

These case improvements in supply chain management within the healthcare organization will not be easy to accomplish, but any organization can make smaller, incremental changes (or more striking changes) to realize a better future. It takes leadership effort, focus, consistency, and a firm foundation to launch a significant improvement effort. It may take capital funds in some areas, such as information systems, software, and training.

Even if an organization is not at present prepared to expend large sums on capital improvements, it can still make considerable inroads toward improving its supply chain operations. Schneller (2006) suggests that there are several keys to better supply chain performance:

- Senior management involvement
- Supply chain optimization as a strategic goal
- Integrated financial and clinical decision making
- Organization cost management focus
- Tracking of performance measures
- End-user accountability for supply cost management
- Physicians' involvement in supply chain activities
- Control of new technology
- Business skills, information, and processes are in place
- Supplier involvement
- Aligned incentives

It is important to note in the above list that improving the supply chain and attaining a more vertically integrated model is often dependent more on leadership's will and less on the availability of capital funds.

To help position the organization at the optimal position in the spectrum, the next chapter introduces the healthcare leader to the concepts of strategic factors and value principles. Proper use of the

Figure 1.6. Sisters of Mercy Health System

In the 1990s, the healthcare supply chain found at Sisters of Mercy Health System was much like those found at many organizations. The fragmented and duplicative systems across Mercy were dependent on six different disparate information technology (IT) materials management software systems; they were unable to negotiate maximized supplier discounts; and they were heavily reliant on outside vendors to help facilitate the management of the health system's supply chains. The opportunity to improve the health system with a total remodeling of the supply chain was identified and pursued.

These realizations resulted in the creation of a new integrated supply chain organization at the system level that better uses available technologies for inventory management and implements supply chain best practices from within and outside the industry. With the creation of a new centralized supply chain, departmental data could then be shared across the system, and Mercy's reliance on outside vendor information was dramatically lessoned.

The creation of the systemwide organization called Resource Optimization Innovation helped consolidate the supply chain throughout Mercy at the corporate level, align major processes utilizing a shared materials management software solution, create an internal GPO, and allow for the enterprise wide management of supply chain distribution and repackaging processes within Mercy. The following initiatives were developed and implemented:

- Creating an internally owned and managed repackaging and distribution facility, the Consolidated Services Center, resulted in
  1. Improved supply chain responsiveness by better catering to customer hospitals, for example, by improving fill rates by 85 percent to 90 percent over what other distributors achieved; and
  2. Streamlined receiving processes by reducing complexity by 70 percent through combined deliveries of medical/surgical items and pharmaceuticals.
- Standard inventory management metrics, like fill rate percentage, measured departmental and centralized performance.
- An internal truck fleet provided more timely deliveries to facilities and improved cost savings by approximately $3 million annually by eliminating third-party markup fees and purchasing directly from manufacturers.
- Bulk purchasing and contracting for economies of scope and scale were made standard procedure.
- Work continues to improve the management of supply chain operations. Furthering currently standardized warehousing practices by focusing on dock-to-bedside practices of the supply chain, Mercy is tackling charge-capture practices, local inventory management processes, and supply-related general ledger design; creating (when applicable) standard operating procedures; and utilizing more extensive supply chain metrics.

  The recently redesigned supply chain has served as a springboard and reinforcement for other functional areas, such as clinical, finance, and revenue, to recognize the inherent value of standardized processes and the efficiencies of consolidation. The launching and second iteration of supply chain-related improvements and efficiency realization serves as the groundwork for establishing a culture of continuous change at Mercy. Clearly, working together across the various functional areas, within the framework of standard files, helping design both clinically and supply chain friendly processes and systems, will create a value-seeking culture that is flexible and ready for change.

Source: Adopted from McCurry et al. 2005.

strategic factors and value principles will enable the improvement and strengthening of the healthcare supply chain, and thus will return greater value in the care delivery process, through efficient use of resources, improved patient care and safety, and improved stakeholder satisfaction.

REFERENCES

Caudle, A. 2006. "Transforming American Healthcare Through Supply Chain Excellence." Panel discussion, Transforming American Healthcare National Symposium, Phoenix, AZ, March 23.

Conway, K. 2006. "Transforming American Healthcare Through Supply Chain Excellence." Panel discussion, Transforming American Healthcare National Symposium, Phoenix, AZ, March 23.

Corry, A., G. Ledlow, and S. Shockley. 2005. "Designing the Standard for a Healthy Supply Chain." In *Achieving Supply Chain Excellence Through Technology (ASCET)*, Vol. 7, 199–202. San Francisco: Montgomery Research.

Freiherr, G. 1996. "The Coming Supply Chain Revolution." *Medical Device & Diagnostic Industry*. [Online article; retrieved 4/26/06.] http://www.devicelink.com/mddi/archive/96/05/009.html.

McCurry, M., V. Moore, G. Kane, and G. Ledlow. 2005. Sisters of Mercy Supply Chain Summit, Branson, MO, October 20–21.

National Patient Safety Foundation (NPSF). 2000. "Agenda for Research and Development in Patient Safety." [Online information; retrieved 4/19/06.] http://www.npsf.org.

Schneller, E. 2006. "Transforming American Healthcare Through Supply Chain Excellence." Panel discussion Transforming American Healthcare National Symposium, Phoenix, AZ, March 23.

CHAPTER 2

Framework for Internal Strategic Decisions

The first responsibility of a leader is to define reality. The last is to say thank you.

—Max DePree

This chapter discusses the supply chain strategic factors and value principles that allow for improved internal strategic decision making. Strategic factors relate generally to the resources that exist currently within an organization, although they can also include resources that could be brought together within a very short and reasonable time frame. A strategic factor assessment tool is provided later in the chapter to help gauge an organization's readiness to improve its supply chain system. ▶

Value principles relate to the operating assumptions and concepts that should be kept in mind as a team works to improve its supply chain system. There are seven strategic factors, all of which can be considered internal to the organization. There are ten value principles discussed in this book: the first eight can be considered internal to the organization, and the last two are externally oriented. This chapter discusses the seven strategic factors and the first eight (internal) value principles. The two external value principles are discussed in Chapter 3. The objective is to establish an organization that is best poised and able to improve and mature its supply chain, based on predetermined goals set by leadership.

SUPPLY CHAIN STRATEGIC FACTORS

The strategic factors are discussed in order of importance. Each strategic factor builds on the previous factor, so they are strongly linked. Strategic factors should be culturally significant within the organization. In addition, they are both tangible and intangible in that strong factors influence good supply chain decisions that are focused on improving patient care and safety,

physician and staff satisfaction, and financial performance. These factors form a base for a solid foundation.

Strategic Factor 1: Information System Usefulness, Electronic Purchasing, and Integration

Good data working in good systems create information that can be turned into knowledge for decision support, decision making, and action. Supply chain information systems should be integrated with the major functions of finance, clinic operations, cost accounting, and revenue in such a way that the healthcare team can speak the same language, use integrative data for joint analyses, make effective decisions, and present individual and aggregated data on transactions. Electronic purchasing significantly reduces errors and discrepancies, especially with use of an electronic catalog.

Strategic Factor 2: Leadership Supply Chain Expertise

Every leader in the organization should have a working understanding of the supply chain's strategic and operational fundamentals to find areas of improvement and to have the ability, as a team, to implement good ideas. This must include the chief executive officer, chief operating officer, chief financial officer, and chief information officer. Each member of the leadership team must talk the same language, which does not happen by itself. Indeed, the language of supply chain is often largely foreign to clinicians, financial staff, and administration. A good exercise to highlight this point would be to simply gather five supply items commonly used in the facility and to ask different people on the team for the items' names, the units of measure, and the use of the items. The odds are great that very different answers will be given (and yet all the answers may be correct in the functional context of the team member). Remember, creating a common language takes effort and a cross-fertilization of contexts and understanding among all team members.

Strategic Factor 3: Supply Chain Expenditures

The more a healthcare organization spends, the greater its power in the marketplace to negotiate price, service, quality, and payment terms. This allows the organization

leverage in the marketplace. It is critical to understand the composition of supply chain expenditures. The medical/surgical and pharmaceutical items' costs (cost of item multiplied by volume) are relatively easy to compute and understand. More difficult costs associated with the supply chain are storage and holding costs (to include facility space and the opportunity cost of the space), transportation costs, inventory management costs, information system costs attributed to supply chain activities, and personnel costs (supply chain and non–supply chain personnel costs of dollars and time). Understanding expenditures and where they accrue are valuable factors in wise decision making.

Strategic Factor 4: Level of Surgeon and Physician Collaboration

The greater the level of surgeon and physician collaboration with leadership (a strategic issue) and the supply chain management team (an operational issue), the greater an organization's ability to compress high-cost and high-volume supplies into one or two manufacturers' supply item lines and thus improve bargaining leverage.

Strategic Factor 5: Level of Nurse and Clinical Staff Collaboration

The greater the level of nurse and clinician collaboration with leadership (a strategic issue) and the supply chain management team (an operational issue), the greater an organization's ability to compress high-cost and high-volume supplies into one or two manufacturers' supply item lines and thus improve bargaining leverage.

Strategic Factor 6: Leadership Team's Political and Social Capital

The ability and willingness of leadership to positively influence and guide the foregoing five items is directly related to the likelihood of success. Creating an expectation; developing a structure of performance, motivation, and incentives; and guiding the organization to meet its goals are at the heart of this factor.

Strategic Factor 7: Availability of Capital Funds

The more capital funds that are available, the greater the ability of an organization to purchase the necessary information systems and to vertically integrate (or keep in-house)

key components of the supply chain. Of course, this should be done as a result of a thorough business case analysis.

Assessment and Scoring of Strategic Factors

Assess your organization's strategic factors using the scale provided in Figure 2.1. The scale runs from one to ten, with one indicating great insufficiency and ten indicating great sufficiency. Do not think hard about each score. Use what first comes to mind to help ensure a fair assessment.

For any strategic factor with a score of four and below, considerable work is needed to attain improvement. Scores between four and seven show a moderate level of potential to improve the supply chain and to implement the supply chain value principles, while scores above seven indicate a solid foundation to improve the organization's supply chain. The strategic factors enable the value prinicples to be better realized. The greater the score for each of the above strategic factors that an organization enjoys, the greater the potential to positively implement the supply chain value principles and to improve the operation.

SUPPLY CHAIN VALUE PRINCIPLES

Value principles are "practice guidelines" for organizational supply chain management and operations.

The strategic factors enable the value principles to be better realized. The greater each strategic factor, the greater the potential to positively implement the supply chain value principles and to

Figure 2.1. Strategic Factor Assessment Tool

Scale of 1 to 10 (10 represents maximum, current sufficiency).
Place an X to assess the organization's current levels of the following:

	1	2	3	4	5	6	7	8	9	10
Example							X			
Information system usefulness, electronic purchasing, and integration										
Leadership supply chain expertise										
Supply chain expenditures										
Level of surgeon and physician collaboration										
Level of nurse and clinical staff collaboration										
Leadership team's political and social capital										
Availability of capital funds										

Work to improve	Moderate potential for success	Good potential for success

improve the operation. Eight internal value principles are discussed, while two external principles are presented in Chapter 3. Each value principle is presented in Table 2.1, which shows the linkages to the strategic factors; two checks (✓ ✓) represent a strong relationship, while one check (✓) represents a moderate relationship for each value principle.

Value Principle 1: Be the Master of the Data (Item, Purchasing History, and Vendor Files)

Credible data that are useful for decision making are paramount to optimizing the supply chain operation. The item and vendor files feed into the purchasing history files (which are essential for departmental analysis of high cost

Table 2.1. Influence of Strategic Factors on Internal Value Principles

Value Principles	Strategic Factors						
	Information system usefulness, electronic purchasing, and integration	Leadership supply chain expertise	Supply chain expenditures	Level of surgeon and physician collaboration	Level of nurse and clinical staff collaboration	Leadership team's political and social capital	Availability of capital funds
Be the master of the data	✓ ✓			✓			✓
Clinical staff should focus on clinical decisions and patient care	✓	✓		✓ ✓	✓ ✓		
Follow the supply items that bring in revenue	✓ ✓	✓	✓	✓	✓ ✓	✓	✓
Increase staff knowledge of supply chain operations		✓ ✓	✓			✓	

Note: Two checks (✓ ✓) represent a strong relationship, while one check (✓) displays a moderate relationship for each value principle.

Value Principles	Strategic Factors						
	Information system usefulness, electronic purchasing, and integration	Leadership supply chain expertise	Supply chain expenditures	Level of surgeon and physician collaboration	Level of nurse and clinical staff collaboration	Leadership team's political and social capital	Availability of capital funds
Determine item, source, contract, and compliance targets for supply chain items of high cost and high volume	✓ ✓	✓	✓	✓ ✓	✓ ✓	✓ ✓	
Develop, standardize, and use supply chain metrics for quality, process, cost, and revenue production	✓ ✓	✓ ✓	✓	✓	✓	✓ ✓	
Develop supply chain goals and objectives by service line for medical/surgical items and pharmaceuticals	✓	✓ ✓	✓	✓	✓	✓	
Structure deliberate short-term and long-term supply chain strategic and operational models	✓	✓ ✓	✓			✓	✓ ✓

Note: Two checks (✓ ✓) represent a strong relationship, while one check (✓) displays a moderate relationship for each value principle.

and high volume). The cleaner and more precise the data, the better the information. This is also critical for selling tracing reports externally, which are used by distributors and manufacturers to do analyses and pay sales representatives the appropriate commissions.

Data must be integrated and standardized (to a high level) across multiple functions, such as finance, revenue generation, and clinical and supply chain systems. This standardization enables, although it does not necessarily create, an "apples to apples" comparison capability to assist in analysis and decision support. The same department names and codes should be used across the systems. If the organization already has a systemwide, multifunctional platform, it is ahead of most healthcare organizations. Consistent supply item names, units of measure, and descriptions should be used across the system and maintained with vigor. Data in the information system must be usable by all functional areas. This is easier said than done, considering the problems of different language and needs of clinicians compared to supply chain managers. All parties must come together to reach agreement, but the bias must be toward the improved

delivery of care rather than the perceived administrative necessities.

All patient-specific chargeable supply items must link consistently across the master item file (the file that contains all items in the supply chain used by your organization) to the charge description master and billing codes. These files and interface links must be managed and corrected continously. This is not only good for data purposes, but also to show systemic compliance with fraud and abuse regulations.

Value Principle 2: Clinical Staff Should Focus on Clinical Decisions and Patient Care

The goal of minimizing supply chain tasks for clinicians and maximizing the effectiveness of their clinical work should be strongly considered. There will always be some level of clinician involvement in supply chain operations, but that time should be efficiently spent. Each organization must determine the appropriate amount of clinician time spent on supply chain tasks.

Every leader in the organization should have a working understanding of the supply chain strategic and operational fundamentals, as well as the importance of being supportive of clinical decision making and patient care. All managers of the organization should appreciate the impact supply chain operations have on all aspects of healthcare delivery and resource management. For example, approximately 15 percent of a nurse's time is spent on supply chain tasks (Friesen 2004). For an entry-level nurse, this equates to over $4,500 per year in supply chain costs attributed to activities such as replenishment, restocking, and supply-item charge-capture tasks. Reducing the supply chain burden on clinicians improves patient safety, efficacy, and satisfaction, as well as enhances clinician satisfaction. In the short term, this may represent a cost shift, and perhaps even a cost addition, by virtue of the need to hire supply chain technicians to replace the supply chain work done by clinicians. In the long run, however, this can provide a significant savings in labor without reducing patient care quality (and can actually enhance patient care).

It is appropriate for some clinician time to be spent on supply chain operations tasks. For example, it is important to involve clinical staff in item selection and contract compliance issues, but they should not be burdened with day-to-day supply chain tasks that can be moved

to less clinically trained staff. Likewise, it is important to minimize supply-item charge-capture time (for items that can be charged separately to a patient's bill) for clinicians by using such modern marvels as smart IT, smart bar-coding technology, radio frequency tagging, and integrated documentation. The bottom line is that with the help of advanced technology, the clinician spends less time in documenting and working with charge-capture processes.

Value Principle 3: Follow the Supply Items that Bring in Revenue (Physically and Electronically)

All supplies that can be billed to the third-party payer or the patient must have positive control and visibility throughout the life cyle of the supply item. Managers throughout the organization should appreciate that all billable supplies (those supplies that can be individually billed to a patient) are tracked and managed in the general information system, as well as by good inventory and revenue charge-capture procedures. A focus on supply items charge-capture processes can improve supply charge-capture rates, often from 50 percent to 90 percent, and thus can substantially improve the bottom line. Also, with aggressive management and data awareness of revenue/charge-capture items, the greater the visibility of supply item volume. The more an organization spends on particular items, the greater its power in the marketplace for negotiating pricing, service, quality, and payment terms.

Value Principle 4: Increase Staff Knowledge of Supply Chain Operations

The leadership team's ability to optimize the supply chain is directly related to its knowledge levels and the importance the senior leader puts on the goal. A positive message of executive-level support can be transmitted by making the supply chain manager an executive in the administrative suite. Begin to educate other leaders and managers on the importance of the supply chain, both strategically and operationally.

Value Principle 5: Determine Item, Source, Contract, and Compliance Targets for Supply Chain Items of High Cost and High Volume

For the healthcare organization to reap the benefits of volume discount pricing and improved service levels, identifying high-cost and high-volume items is essential. These are the supply items where the most negotiated gains can be achieved with suppliers. The following outlines a sequence of tasks to achieve better pricing and service for the highest-cost supply items:

- Using purchasing history files, determine the top high-volume and high-price supply items in both medical/surgical and pharmaceutical areas.
- Involve surgeons, physicians, nurses, and other clinicians in the selection process to move purchases for a particular item to one or two manufacturers. Negotiate a substantially discounted price for the item in exchange for market share (organizational compliance), and monitor the internal compliance rates (compliance is meeting the elements of a negotiated contract). If the supplier gives a 15 percent discount for an 80 percent usage rate for its product(s), then compliance is meeting the 80 percent or better usage rate in the healthcare organization for the contracted supplier's product(s).
- Reward compliance and above-compliance goal attainment by departments. Determine which items are high cost and high volume; which items have high

physician preference (surgical gloves, for example); which items have high nurse preference (IV start kits, for example), also called clinical commodities; and those items with high staff preference, also called commodities (toilet paper and copier paper, for example) for each service line. Look for consolidation/ standardization opportunities for each item type by service-line groupings, such as orthopedics, cardiology, skilled nursing, and so on. From there, organizationwide consolidation/standardization of an item can occur. It is possible to save as much as 20 percent by consolidating to one vendor and to achieve high compliance rates by utilizing that vendor's products to a high degree (80 percent to 90 percent) for a service line such as cardiology within the cardiac rhythm management supply chain. Start with supply items in high-cost and high-volume service lines.

Value Principle 6: Develop, Standardize, and Use Supply Chain Metrics for Quality, Process, Cost, and Revenue Production

It is important to develop standard metrics for the supply chain with regard to service, quality, and cost, so that they include adjusted patient-day supply cost, supply transaction cost, high-volume and high-cost trending, service rates (fulfillment, back order, and "fill or kill"), and quality measures. Have these metrics reported and published regularly (at least monthly). Metrics should include timeliness, accuracy, and fullfillment rates for service quality; but for financial tracking, you should include the following:

Cost performance measures: A single method with specific measures for evaluating supply expense should be identified and used consistently. Examples of measures include: 1. Supply cost as a percentage of net revenue, 2. Supply cost as a percentage of total expense, 3. Supply cost per adjusted patient day, and 4. Supply cost per adjusted discharge.

Because no single method is universally accepted as the "best," many hospitals and integrated delivery systems use a mix of these metrics, applied consistently. The organizations track these performance measures over time as a way to manage their supply chain expenses. Just as important as the choice of which combination of metrics to use, however, is the selection of peer hospitals or IDSs (Integrated Delivery Systems) to benchmark against. To level the playing field, the case mix index is often used in conjunction with the performance measures. Unfortunately, use of the case mix index sometimes compounds the problem of true comparability because the Medicare case weight was designed as a means to relate resource consumption among different patient types (or Diagnosis Related Groups—DRGs), rather than as a predictor of actual supply and pharmacy cost utilization. For example, DRG 79 (Respiratory Infections, w/CC) has a Medicare case weight of 1.58 and an average direct supply cost per case of $1,000. Conversely, DRG 250 (Cervical Spine Fusion without CC) has a Medicare case weight of 1.62 and an average direct supply cost of $4,000 per case. Thus, although the Medicare case weights are almost identical, the supply costs per procedure differ by nearly 400 percent. This significant difference between a DRG that reflects a medical condition and a DRG that reflects a surgical procedure underscores the importance of selecting the correct peer group for supply performance metrics. If the facility is driven largely by surgical procedures, one should compare the supply chain performance metrics with those of other procedure-driven hospitals, not of hospitals with primarily medical populations.

The goal of measurement should not be to simply track absolute line-item savings in a given supply category. Rather, the focus should be on relating supply and other expenses to revenues, to determine, for example, the degree to which the facility achieves total cost savings by procedure or service line (Ballard 2005).

Measuring the rates of supply chain service is extremely important as part of documenting of overall customer service. It is important to be able to identify when costs are incurred for the purpose of improving supply chain service. Quantifiable evidence such as this can be used to either support or disprove the effectiveness of the expenditure. It is also necessary to understand the monetary value of the perceived satisfaction to determine the effectiveness of the expenditure in this area. Two of the major metrics used to determine customer service levels are that of fulfillment rates and back order versus fill or kill (if item is not in stock, the order is killed) occurrences. Standardized quality metrics can help quantify process efficiency. It is imperative that these metrics are reported frequently and consistently to facilitate trending and to measure change over time.

Value Principle 7: Develop Supply Chain Goals and Objectives by Service Line for Medical/Surgical Items and Pharmaceuticals

Starting with the greatest areas of promise (such as surgery, cardiac catheterization laboratory, pharmacy, radiology, and laboratory), have each service line set goals and objectives for supply chain optimization in the areas of service, cost, and quality. Be sure to include a goal related to reducing stored inventory. Much of the stored inventories within departments are unmanaged; just consider how stored inventories tend to vanish just before a Joint Commission survey! Have the goals and objectives be a part of the operational plan that rolls up into the organizational strategic plan,

and report on progress at regular intervals.

To set, report progress toward, and achieve goals, seek "champions" among the physicians and nurses. Use existing organizational structures, such as the pharmaceutical and therapeutics committee, the capital committee, and so forth. Alternatively, establish new groups to focus on service line problems related to supply chain issues. For example, one organization invited physicians, laboratory managers, and administrators to serve on a committee to help analyze service lines with negative or narrow margins. It was discovered that too many all-inclusive laboratory tests (called Chemical 20s, or Chem 20s) were being ordered by physicians. The committee recommended that Chemical 7s, Chemical 5s, and a few specific tests would become the preferred standard. This recommendation was adopted by the physicians and other clinicians. The system enjoyed an approximate 20 percent decrease of reagent costs as a result; clinicians monitoring the change over time determined that there was no loss of quality in patient care, but they happily noticed faster test results for their patients.

Value Principle 8: Structure Deliberate Short-Term and Long-Term Supply Chain Strategic and Operational Models

Leaders are vital to building a strategic foundation for the supply chain, so they must deliberately select and work toward creating the culture, model, and operational parameters which with to manage by the supply chain. Each organization will be different as needs, situational issues, and level of strategic factors differ. So, each leadership team at each organization must determine their supply chain elements. Following is a suggested sequence of tasks:

- Conduct a thorough business analysis of the organization's supply chain operation in terms of service, cost, quality, satisfaction, and opportunities.
- Make a conscious decision about the organization's supply chain structure for the short term and long term.

- Budget for and implement the organization's plan based on a thorough business analysis and on the leadership team's commitment.

SUMMARY

This chapter focused on strategic factors and value principles to enable and facilitate an improved supply chain from an internal perspective. This framework can foster an improved infrastructure and internal strategic decision making by senior leaders with regard to supply chain management. Table 2.1 illustrates the linkage of the most important enabling strategic factors to the internal value principles.

Internal value principles greatly empower external action and capabilities. Two important value principles remain, and these relate to important external issues in strategic planning for improved supply chain management.

REFERENCES

Ballard, R. 2005. "Strategic Supply Cost Management Physician Preference Without Deference: Adopting a Strategic Approach to Managing Supply Chain Costs Can Lead to a Productive Dialogue Between Physicians and Financial Leaders." *Healthcare Financial Management* 59 (4): 78–80, 82, 84.

Friesen, S. 2004. "The Canadian Healthcare Supply Chain Landscape." Healthcare Supply Chain Summit, Toronto, Ontario, Canada, September 22.

CHAPTER 3

Framework for External Strategic Decisions

A leader takes people where they want to go. A great leader takes people where they don't necessarily want to go but ought to be.

—Rosalynn Carter

This chapter focuses on two additional value principles (that is, operating assumptions and concepts that should be kept in mind as a team works to improve its supply chain system) that are external in nature. The perspectives of the various players in the supply chain process are reviewed. That is, the mission, process, goals, and incentives of the stakeholders in the supply chain are presented. The stakeholders include the manufacturers, distributors, GPOs, transportation organizations, and healthcare providers. Finally, tips are provided on how to manage the external relationships in the supply chain. ▶

TWO EXTERNAL VALUE PRINCIPLES

Both internal and external value principles depend on strategic factors. However, external principles are also dependent on organizations external to the healthcare organization. Leaders in healthcare organizations must understand the interaction, dependency, and value of the relationship for each significant external organization associated with the supply chain. The externally oriented value principles emphasize the importance of qualifying and quantifying supply chain relationships. These value principles offer a process and a system to qualify and quantify external stakeholders associated with the supply chain. Table 3.1 illustrates

Table 3.1. Influence of Strategic Factors on External Value Principles

Value Principles	Information system usefulness, electronic purchasing, and integration	Leadership supply chain expertise	Supply chain expenditures	Level of surgeon and physician collaboration	Level of nurse and clinical staff collaboration	Leadership team's political and social capital	Availability of capital funds
	Strategic Factors						
Decide which external manufacturers and/or distributors the organization wants to work with directly—and remember the 80/20 rule	✓ ✓	✓	✓ ✓	✓	✓	✓	
Manage external group purchasing, distribution, and transportation partners/organizations	✓	✓	✓ ✓				

Note: Two checks (✓ ✓) represent a strong relationship, while one check (✓) represents a moderate relationship for each value principle.

the linkage and dependency of the following two value principles on the strategic factors.

Value Principle 9: Decide Which External Manufacturers and/or Distributors the Organization Wants to Work with Directly—And Remember the "80/20 Rule"

Approximately 80 percent of the dollar value of purchases comes from or through 20 percent of the manufacturers or distributors (also called vendors) in a typical healthcare organization. It is important to select those supply items that are high volume and/or high priced and to negotiate with one or two of the manufacturers or vendors for discounted pricing for that supply item or items. The goal should be to reduce cost and improve service to the organization through compression (that is, moving from several suppliers to one or two suppliers for supply items of a certain type or line). Cost reduction is achieved through negotiation based on utilization percentage. Compression, or narrowing suppliers to one or two for a particular supply item, and the utilization of that supply item based on a negotiated pricing

structure (utilization percentage, which is usually 75 percent to 90 percent) garner steep pricing discounts and increased rebates. How well the organization complies with utilization contract terms for those negotiated supply items is the fundamental tenet of contract compliance (also known as organizational compliance) from a supply chain perspective.

The Health Industry Group Purchasing Association (HIGPA) is a good source of information related to the supply chain patterns of various GPOs, especially as they relate to contractual compliance:

> While the HIGPA report documents the many products and services that GPOs offer their members, it reveals that GPO members purchase a significant proportion of their goods through direct negotiations with suppliers. These observations add credence to the contention that today's most pressing supply chain issue, for suppliers as well as for group purchasing organizations, is contract compliance by members. In multi-hospital systems, the purchasing function continues to have the focus at the individual hospital level, with inconsistent

approaches toward system-wide corporate purchasing and negotiation (Schneller 2000).

Compliance by healthcare providers brings leverage to the negotiating table. The following tenets help providers achieve compression and contract compliance:

- Involve surgeons, physicians, nurses, and clinical staff in selection and compliance-setting tasks to improve satisfaction and compliance.
- Focus on surgery (cardiac rhythm management and orthopedics, for example), cardiac catheterization laboratory, pharmacy, radiology, and laboratory as excellent starting points for the biggest return on effort that will positively affect the bottom line.

Value Principle 10: Manage External Group Purchasing, Distribution, and Transportation Partners/Organizations

Select the most important external relationships of your supply chain and manage those connections. Starting with the previously mentioned 80/20 rule, analyze the organization's purchasing history by manufacturer and/or vendor to identify the top 20 percent of manufacturers and vendors the healthcare organization uses. Plans concerning compression and the value of each external relationship can be determined from this simple list. Ways to evaluate relationships with external organizations are discussed later in this chapter.

Concurrently, determine the organization's needs and discuss these needs with manufacturers and/or vendors. Use the same method of determining the top 20 percent of supply items by cost (high cost and/or volume), and identify needs and expectations regarding supply item quality, delivery timeliness, quantity, and any criteria important to the healthcare organization. If the analysis is done correctly, both the top manufacturers or vendors and the top supply items should have considerable overlap; this will direct focus and effort to improving the supply chain from the external organization perspective.

These external value principles will help improve the organization's supply chain operation and will help the organization reach its vision of a better supply chain environment. More discussion about external issues follows in this chapter.

THE STAKEHOLDERS' PERSPECTIVE

To be able to make quality decisions about your own organization's supply chain, it is important to understand the various stakeholders and their respective mission, process, goals, and incentives within the chain. This section provides a summary of the mission, process, goals, and incentives of external stakeholders of the healthcare supply chain: manufacturers, distributors, GPOs, transportation organizations, and healthcare providers.

Manufacturers

MISSION. The general mission of the manufacturer is to produce quality, sellable products that incur the smallest cost of production, while enjoying the highest profit margin possible. By minimizing the overall management and production costs of the items, the manufacturer is able to increase its realized profit margin. For example, by reducing the number of physical locations to which items must be delivered, or by minimizing the number of different units of measure that are available for sale, the manufacturer is able to streamline production and minimize expense.

PROCESS. The manufacturer strives to use sophisticated IT that provides real-time manufacturing data as it receives raw materials and products and transforms them into sellable products. The manufacturer generally produces sellable products in batches and attempts to limit the amount of production setup and overhead costs, as well as assembly "dead time." Batch production at times produces a significant supply surplus of the manufacturer's most profitable items, despite limited need, which can often be pushed on the distributor. Using sequencing, timing, and forecasting techniques, the manufacturer manages production in the most profitable manner possible.

GOALS AND INCENTIVES. The goal of the manufacturer is to sell as many of their most profitable manufactured products as possible, while incurring the least amount of cost and thus generating the greatest amount of profit. By using top-moving products to negotiate for the purchase of its entire line of supplies and products, the manufacturer attempts to expand the breadth of its supply and the product line items sold to distributors and providers.

Distributors

MISSION. The distributor's principal mission is to become an integral and irreplaceable middle resource between the manufacturer and the provider (healthcare customer). By supplying what is perceived as a needed and otherwise unavailable service, the distributor remains a necessary player. The distributor achieves quantities of scale that allow it to be profitable from minimal markups on each individual item. The distributor attempts to sell items to health systems based on profit margins rather than the health system's needs.

PROCESS. The basic process of the distributor is to receive bulk inventory from the manufacturer and repackage and redistribute the items to many healthcare providers. The distributor strives to maintain as little inventory as possible, while "turning" the inventory as frequently as possible. Turning the inventory is defined as selling and removing existing inventory with new inventory; essentially, it is throughput of the entire portfolio of supply items. Turning the inventory frequently, such as weekly or monthly, is the preference. The distributor, in essence, adds an incremental charge to the cost of its products for the service of delivering the products. The distributor is perceived to be an essential component of most contemporary healthcare delivery systems.

GOALS AND INCENTIVES. The distributor's goal is to become as profitable as possible by selling the products with the highest profit margin to the provider (consumer) in an expedient and low-cost manner. By quick turnaround of item inventory (turning) and keeping storage levels as low as possible, the retaining inventory costs are minimized. By delivering to the fewest locations and selling all products within its inventory (regardless of provider demand), the distributor's profits are magnified. This sometimes creates situations in which the distributor pushes items onto the provider, however.

The distributor's goal is to be perceived as a "one-stop shop" by the provider and to have a diverse line of products that meets all or most of the needs of the provider. The distributor attempts to create a trusting and ongoing relationship with the provider, in part by maintaining appropriate fill rates of products and by complying with timely delivery requirements agreed to with the provider. In addition to simply distributing products, many distributors further their broad service line of products by becoming a self-manufacturer of items or a repackager of items that can be positioned for the "bait and switch." This is similar to the Wal-Mart "generic" brand or the brands of other chain retailers; the retailer's brand items (retailer-packaged items, many times by the same manufacturer of the brand name product) are shelved next to "brand name" products. This ability to supplement or switch products with internally produced or repackaged items allows the distributor even greater profitability.

In short, the distributor attempts to serve as an intermediary, communicator, and sales agent between the manufacturer and the provider. The distributor can charge a markup on items for its services by virtue of providing repackaging, quantity inventorying, and redistribution. By maintaining key data related to product demand, the distributor can sell or offer valuable information to the manufacturer for future production determination. The distributor strives to place itself as a valuable provider of information to both the manufacturer and the provider, because product consumption data are otherwise not easily attained without the distributor's efforts.

Group Purchasing Organizations

MISSION. The GPO's mission is to increase its membership of providers, while negotiating the best purchasing prices possible from distributors and manufacturers. The GPO seeks to gain greater volume leverage and negotiation power with distributors by attaining an expanding base of providers (members). Serving as a contracting and information-collection intermediary between distributors and providers of healthcare, GPOs offer a wide breadth of contracting services negotiated as a third party.

PURPOSE. The GPO seeks to provide competitive pricing for its providers, while serving as an outsourced supply chain purchasing contract service. Because it has huge purchasing power based on the collective providers' purchasing power, the GPO is positioned to contract for discounted purchase prices. Two or more distributors can compete with each other for the loyalty of GPO providers by providing excellent communication/feedback and other informational services, as well as by touting preferred pricing contracts that have been achieved.

Goals and Incentives. The goal of the GPO is to be recognized in the market as having the greatest purchasing power, based on size and number of providers. By attempting to be perceived as a necessary intermediary negotiator between the distributor and the provider, the GPO attempts to negotiate items that are most profitable to itself—and not necessarily items that the endbuyers are asking it to negotiate. It is important to note that many GPOs are also starting to participate in freight management contracting services as a method of diversification.

Transportation Organizations

Mission and Purpose. The transportation organization's mission and purpose is to move products along the supply chain, ultimately to the provider healthcare organizations, in a reliable, cost-effective manner.

Goals and Incentives. Freight management and distribution costs borne by the distributor or manufacturer are usually absorbed within the price of goods and are eventually passed along to the healthcare provider. It is often difficult then to differentiate the actual costs of the movement of the item from the charge for the actual item and other fees.

The manufacturers and distributors, having managed the freight costs of items for many years, have actually found the management of costs associated with freight management to be financially beneficial to their organizations' revenue. Because they receive volume discounts from major freight managers (UPS, FedEx, etc.) that are most often not fully passed on to the buyer, the difference between the actual cost of shipment and the charged shipment fees serves as a profitable arena for most distributors (Neil 2005).

Thus, the manufacturer and distributor have an incentive to continue to determine the freight amounts, bundle the freight costs in the overall item cost, and obtain volume discounts for shipping that are not passed on to the buyer, regardless of how the supply items are transported to the healthcare provider.

Healthcare Providers

Mission. For purposes of this discussion, the provider of healthcare services (health systems and hospital operations) is considered to be the health system and/or the individual hospitals that make up the health system. The provider seeks to minimize costs and maintain the lowest inventory levels possible, while having sufficient products available for consumption when needed. By being creative and adapting successes from other industries, the provider's operational departments attempt to be more efficient and cost-effective, while maintaining a predetermined level of care and hospitality service for their end-user patient-customers.

The recognized core function of the provider is quality healthcare delivery. Unfortunately, logistical efficiency and operational effectiveness are not usually considered core functions. Because of this, healthcare providers typically lack the necessary modern technology to maintain an effective supply chain system. Saddled with manual or outdated processes, the provider's departments are often challenged with the reality of "just getting it done" in an environment of limited funding.

PURPOSE. The provider of healthcare services strives to ensure that those delivering services to patients are given what they need and when they really need it. A continuing dilemma within healthcare is the perceived need at the departmental level to stock items unofficially in various cabinets, closets, and other clandestine locations.

GOALS AND INCENTIVES. A principal goal of the healthcare provider is to provide its services effectively and efficiently. It is important to note that services can be provided internally or externally (by an outsourced entity). An important goal is to create a relationship of trust with the end user, which can be accomplished by dealing with all suppliers that provide quality service. It is vital for the overall success of the supply chain to work with organizations that have built reputations of reliability over time.

Other key goals include product standardization and consolidation of the number of unique items available within the system. This can reduce the operational costs of the provider's supply chain management activities. An organization should strive to minimize the number of individual SKUs (a unique supply or pharmaceutical item that is stored and managed as inventory) that need to be managed, which would allow for minimization of overall inventory and increased shelf space. Increased shelf space can permit greater volume of certain items to take advantage of discounts on certain items as the discounts become available. By minimizing the number of unique manufacturers and distributors from which products are purchased, a more relationship-driven, volume-based process can occur, with lower overhead management costs. The principle is simple: The less material to manage, the easier and more cost-effective the processes are in the operation.

Customized solutions are needed to effectively manage various specific high-need areas, such as preoperative care and cardiac catheterization laboratories. An organization can use collaboration and incentives to help ensure contractual compliance and to prevent the unwanted selling efforts by suppliers that are not preferred.

Table 3.2 provides examples of the different conflicting goals of the

Table 3.2. Healthcare Supply Chain Model Stakeholder Conflicts

Manufacturers want...	Distributors want...	Providers (hospitals and health systems) want...
To reduce costs of production and distribution to enhance margins	To store/carry the fewest number of profitable items possible in the lowest quantities possible	To minimize their purchase points and reduce distribution fees
To produce in large batch sizes to reduce production costs	To be the collector of usage data so that they can sell it to the manufacturer (as sales tracing reports)	To deal with people they can trust
To ship their product to the fewest locations possible	To sell the most profitable products to the customer	To minimize counter-selling efforts of sales representatives in their departments
To ship the product in pallet or truckload quantities	To augment their offering with self-manufactured items that can be positioned for the bait and switch	To reduce the number of items to store, to manage SKUs, and to reduce inventory
To have the customers buy their entire product line exclusively	To have high turnover of their inventory	To be innovative
To have real-time data on how and where their products are being used and in what quantities	To have their customers use them as the one-stop shop for healthcare items and not compete with other distributors for same or similar items	To obtain guarantees on service and product availability

stakeholders of the supply chain, based on the traditional model.

TIPS ON MANAGING EXTERNAL RELATIONSHIPS

Consider doing an assessment of supply chain needs and wants across the organization. Take that information and have the leadership/management of the organization create a document that expresses the organization's must haves, should haves, and would like to haves. From this work, the leadership team will have a platform with which to build relationships with manufacturers, distributors, and others. The next step is to determine how those external partners fit in the organization's relationship model.

Manufacturer and Distributor Evaluations

Not all external relationships are the same. Some are more valuable, and some are potentially more valuable than others. A good exercise, based on the healthcare organization's needs and wants, would be to place existing (and potential or future) external supply chain organizations that have a relationship with the

healthcare organization into four categories: core, developmental, required, and minor.

CORE. The healthcare organization should determine which of its relationships are core. Core relationships are those that have the most likelihood of developing into long-term, value-adding partnerships. Core manufacturers and distributors, therefore, are those that are the most sought-after types of partnerships with whom to engage in business relationships. Because of their potential for developing into long-term relationships that can prove to be beneficial to both parties, they provide high relative value and are highly attractive to providers. The goal is to build or move as many manufacturers/vendors into this category of relationship. From an overall perspective of partnership evaluation, the core relationships are those that should be most heavily sought. Core relationships are strategic and crucial partnerships.

DEVELOPMENTAL. Developmental external relationships are ones in which manufacturers and/or distributors work collaboratively and willingly with the healthcare organization to develop better business partnerships. Currently low in relative value, these developmental relationships offer the potential for improvement because of the attractiveness of the overall relationship to your organization. For example, a manufacturer whose current relationship is providing little value but is attractive because of the partner's willingness to cooperate and to provide better-quality products, packages, or services would be considered developmental. Developmental relationships have potential, with time and continued effort, to develop into core relationships.

REQUIRED. Required relationships have great relative value but fall short of the requisite level of attractiveness to be elevated to a core or developmental relationship. Organizations in the required category have a mutual dependence with the healthcare organization and, at first glance, may seem desirable for a partner. However, for some reason, the relationship is stagnant. Perhaps the values of the two organizations are vastly different, or the manufacturer or distributor is not willing to work with the healthcare organization's

changing needs. Identifying competitors of required category manufacturers and/or distributors is the basic strategy to remedy the unfavorable relationship. By finding other sources or identifying ways to make the relationship more desirable, required partners can be replaced by competitors who could become long-term core partners.

MINOR. Manufacturers and distributors are the least important because of their relatively low overall value and the low attractiveness of the relationship. Minor partners have the potential of desirability, but they are currently providing little benefit to the healthcare organization. A minor relationship, for example, is a manufacturer that is not willing to negotiate better pricing and service, even though several other manufacturers produce the same or similar products. These manufacturers and/or distributors, falling below par in both attractiveness of the relationship and in overall value to the healthcare organization, need to be continuously evaluated. The basic strategy is to either foster the relationship to make it more attractive or to shift business to a different partner that has a higher evaluation. The minor category relationships do not add strategic advantage to your organization. However, they do steal resources (opportunity cost) from the healthcare organization because minor category relationships must still be managed and operationally supported.

It is important to understand how relationships provide value. Being able to quickly identify the most valuable core partners and the least valuable minor partners is an important analysis for strategic development in building a solid supply chain foundation.

Decisions of Involvement with Manufacturers and Distributors

For a long-term strategy, following these simple rules should help the organization structure a plan of action to build, nurture, and maintain core and developmental relationships (Kane 2005), such as the following:

- Focus on significant manufacturer and distributor relationships.
- Build secondary manufacturer relationships.
- Open a discussion with competitors of current manufacturers.

- Evaluate start-up manufacturers for relationship building.

It is also important to know what motivates external partners. These four concerns are paramount to the healthcare organization's external supply chain partners and potential partners:

1. Growth: How big is the potential deal?
2. Market share: Based on the given volume, how much market share does the external partner receive? The basic elements are commitment and ability to deliver on commitment (provider compliance).
3. Length of term: How long can the external partner be assured of this business at the volume and compliance levels committed to by the healthcare organization? External players wish to gain and hold market share as long as possible.
4. Margin: Does the opportunity present itself in a way that allows the external partner to save money and increase margin? (This can include increased quantity per order, increased quantity per ship-to point, and reduced cost of sales).

This chapter has focused on the external strategic decisions that a healthcare organization needs to consider in the quest to improve its supply chain system. Two external value principles were presented. The perspectives of the key stakeholders or partners in the supply chain process were reviewed, and a methodology for evaluating the healthcare organization's relationships with external manufacturers and distributors was described.

The next chapter takes the principles provided thus far and applies them to real-world projects that can enhance any healthcare organization's supply chain management system, with a special emphasis on the improvement of operational and bottom-line performance.

REFERENCES

Kane, G. 2006. "Transforming American Healthcare Through Supply Chain Excellence." Panel discussion, Transforming American Healthcare National Symposium, Phoenix, AZ, March 23.

Neil, R. 2005. "Planes, Trains, and Automobiles." *Materials Management in Healthcare* 14 (2): 16–19.

Schneller, E. 2000. *The Value of Group Purchasing in the Health Care Supply Chain.* Tempe, AZ: School of Health Administration and Policy, College of Business, Arizona State University.

CHAPTER 4

Opportunities to Improve Operation and Bottom Line

An empowered organization is one in which individuals have the knowledge, skill, desire, and opportunity to personally succeed in a way that leads to collective organizational success.

—Stephen R. Covey, Principle-Centered Leadership

Healthcare leadership team members need to understand whether their organization more closely resembles the traditional model or the vertically integrated model of supply chain management, as well as where they would like their organization to be in the next few years. Likewise, team members should understand the value principles behind effective supply chain management and be able to determine the level of development that they would like to see in their strategic factors. This chapter suggests a series of projects that can help your healthcare organization gain incremental victories, while improving the supply chain management system, the healthcare delivery operation, and the financial bottom line. Each project should be evaluated for prioritization and "worthiness" for your organization. ▶

For each project, the anticipated level of effort, expected impact, action steps, and the project's link to a value principle(s) are presented.

SIX PROJECTS FOR YOUR ORGANIZATION

Project 1: Develop Online Supply Chain Training and User Support Tools

Supporting value principle: Increase staff knowledge of supply chain operations.

Financial impact estimate: Reduce supply chain operation and item cost, across the organization, by 2 percent to 5 percent.

Effort: High
Benefit: High

Cost estimates:
- Adobe Captivate (formerly RoboDemo) software to create flash video courses ($500)
- Supply chain operations expert to create online courses and documentation (250–500 hours)
- Information technology staff to load (4 hours) and support (2 hours per week) courses and documentation on Web server

- Supply chain operations staff member to manage content and live chat sessions (4–8 hours per week)

Description: This project focuses on improving training materials and access to supply chain information, knowledge, skills, and abilities. This could include online 24/7 training with animated courses that incorporate practice tasks and testing, bulletin board for end users to post needed or unneeded items, scheduled chat line with experts available for online discussions, and continuing education credits and defined skill-level paths.

Steps toward action:
1. Purchase and develop software tool or tools.
2. Coordinate with IT department for online use.
3. Coordinate with human resources department for end-user participation history.
4. Create training content, tools, and materials (start simple).
5. Receive leadership approval for process, content, and requirements.

Performance indicators/metrics:

- Volume usage noted through user log

- Staff skill path and levels
- New items added to or obtained from bulletin board
- Participants on scheduled chat

Project 2: Develop Point-of-Use Supply Charge-Capture and Automated Replenishment System with Reconciliation Procedures

Supporting value principles:
- Follow the supply items that bring in revenue.
- Develop, standardize, and use supply chain metrics for quality, process, cost, and revenue production.
- Develop supply chain goals and objectives by service line for medical/surgical items and pharmaceuticals.

Financial impact estimate: Reduce costs by 1 percent to 2 percent, attributed to charge capture and supplies replenishment. Potentially increase charge-capture efficiency (revenue for supply items that can be charged to the payer; many organizations have a supply-item charge-capture rate of 50 percent to 70 percent) by 20 percent to 30 percent.

Effort: High
Benefit: High

Cost estimates:
- Purchase of a technology solution, including hardware, software, and training (approximately $750–$1,250 per hospital bed)
- Potential modifications of storage locations and equipment (situation specific)

Description: In this project, you will implement the latest technology (such as bar-code scanning), allowing for point-of-use capture of supply consumption. This knowledge of supply usage can automate patient charging, decrease inventory, and automate purchase orders. Using the latest technology allows for easier reconciliation of patient charges for supplies. By comparing supply issues to patient charges, this allows for better management of potential revenues. Develop, communicate, and implement clear processes to ensure compliance and control based on selected point of use system.

Steps toward action:
1. Document the current and future state processes, as well as the select a vendor solution for implementation:

a. Define best practices in supply charge capture; and

   b. Perform a vendor selection process to choose the best solution.

2. Emphasize clinical end-user work flow and patient care.

3. Adopt a methodology that matches revenue and expense to the cost center that provided patient care.

4. Educate management and staff about the importance of tracked data to maximize revenue capture.

5. Accurately interface or link point-of-use charge-capture system with supply chain system and charge master and billing systems.

Performance indicators/metrics:

- Percent charge-capture rate for chargeable supply items by department:
  - Departmental lost supply charges
  - Patient bill accuracy for supply chargeable items
- Average supply cost per procedure or admitting diagnosis
- Number of stock-outs (when a needed supply item is not available) per department
- Contract usage rates and compliance

Project 3: Develop a Methodology to Support Continuous Product Standardization and Consolidation

Supporting value principles:

- Determine item, source, contract, and compliance targets for supply chain items of high cost and high volume.
- Decide which external manufacturers and/or distributors the organization wants to work with directly—and remember the 80/20 rule.

Financial impact estimate: Reduce total number of suppliers, selecting those with the best core and developmental relationships (and required category relationships, if absolutely necessary), while reducing the total number of different items being managed, to reduce costs of supply items by service line (such as cardiac rhythm management supplies) by 5 percent to 20 percent. Overall, total supply chain savings could reach 5 percent to 9 percent if four or five major service lines adopt and implement this strategy.

Effort: High
Benefit: High

Cost estimates:

- Supply chain representative to design standardization intiative and manage ongoing relationships with manufacturers and distributors (approximately $30,000 per service line)
- Information management staff to perform ongoing analysis identifying like-type items for potential consolidation (2 hours per week) and to perform project effectiveness analysis (2 hours per week) (approximately $15,000 per year per organization, such as a hospital)
- Supply chain representative and clinical staff to manage consolidation efforts (1 hour per week), although this task may be accomplished without additional cost

Description: This project involves agreeing on standardized items and allowing for fewer unique items to be managed from preferred manufacturers and/or distributors (hopefully, core or developmental partners). It is necessary to perform ongoing analysis to determine functional equivalents for commodity items, so that as few supply items are managed as possible. This will allow for greater volume purchasing of a single item and will reduce the overall number of total items needing to be maintained. Greater volume purchases and higher compliance rates (meeting negotiated utilization targets and measurements) will allow for better negotiations with the supplier of the standardized item.

Steps toward action:

1. Perform current-state analysis of functional equivalent items that are being maintained.
2. Determine when and where consolidation and standardization of these items are feasible.
3. Select the appropriate vendors to have an ongoing relationship with and to source these items.
4. Create an education program for clinical managers, showing how consolidation can facilitate volume, which can reduce cost from supplier.
5. Receive clinical buy-in of compliance cost-benefits and leadership approval for process, content, and requirements.

Performance indicators/metrics:

- Consolidated item compliance levels for preferred supplier and nonpreferred suppliers
- Cost savings derived from increased volume of consolidated item purchase

- Total number of managed supply items in stock area and within item file

Project 4: Develop Comprehensive Enhancements to Improve Surgery Inventory Management

Supporting value principles:
- Clinical staff should focus on clinical decisions and patient care.
- Develop supply chain goals and objectives by service line for medical/surgical items and pharmaceuticals.

Financial impact estimate: Increase the capability to perform a true case-cost analysis and demonstrate purchase compliance for preferred supplier items, enabling a 5 percent to 10 percent potential supply cost and management savings within the surgery department.

Effort: High
Benefit: High

Cost estimates:
- Brainstorming session to set compliance goals for both surgical area consumption compliance and supply chain support role (2–4 hours, including preparation time, for approximately $7,500)
- Inventory specialist to make recommendations on inventory reduction, as well as on consolidation and compliance goals (2 hours per week, for approximately $7,000 to $9,000 per year per organization)
- Data analyst to perform a current-state analysis of clinical staff's time commitment to supply-related activities (approximately $3,500 per organization)
- Supply chain operations staff member to manage weekly customer service meetings with surgical staff representatives (2 hours per week, for approximately $10,000 per year per organization)

Description: In this project, an improved understanding can be obtained of how to better manage surgical inventory by formalizing communication via ongoing meetings between the surgical customer department and the supporting supply chain department. One of the intended outcomes of this project is to help the clinicians minimize the amount of time spent performing supply chain tasks and focus more on treating patients. By setting predetermined compliance goals for high-cost and high-volume items, contracting based on consolidation and standardization can be sought. It is vital that both parties participate in ongoing improvement of surgical inventory management, because a great deal of supply cost and revenue is consumed and produced, respectively, within the perioperative area.

Steps toward action:
1. Develop desired metrics.
2. Coordinate with surgery to communicate purpose and desired outcomes.
3. Perform current clinician supply time and high-cost, high-volume supply usage analyses.
4. Identify key participants and schedule ongoing meetings.
5. Receive leadership approval for process, content, and requirements.

Performance indicators/metrics:
- Cost reduction from item consolidation of high-cost and high-volume items
- Clinical staff time spent on supply chain–related tasks
- Number of compliance goals met by both clinical staff and supply chain
- Clinical staff overall program compliance

Project 5: Develop a Model to Support Optimal Product and Vendor Selection

Supporting value principles:
- Determine item, source, contract, and compliance targets for supply chain items of high cost and high volume.
- Decide which external manufacturers and/or distributors the organization wants to work with directly—and remember the 80/20 rule.
- Manage external group purchasing, distribution, and transportation partners/organizations.

Financial impact estimate: Perform continuous product consolidation and standardization with external core and developmental partners that provide the greatest long-term cost benefits, to achieve a 2 percent to 3 percent overall supply chain savings.

Effort: Low
Benefit: Moderate

Cost estimates:
- Development (40 hours) and ongoing management of product consolidation model metrics (3 hours per week, for approximately $8,000–$12,000)

- Development of supplier program to manage vendor performance metrics (16 intial hours and then 2 hours per week, for approximately $5,000–$7,500)

Description: This project includes establishing a program to analyze the desired supplier relationships (core, developmental, required, and minor), along with their levels of compliance, to help optimize desired future working arrangements. By formally evaluating the manufacturer and/or distributors based on the desired levels of service and their ability to meet agreed on commitments, your organization can be better served in the future. Future product-line consolidation and standardization efforts of the organization will be furthered by strategically aligning the manufacturer relationships and by achieving contractual savings with these suppliers. Similarly, the management of external GPOs, distributors, and transportation partners is necessary for furthering the long-term selection of appropriate partners. Utilization of a model to aid in the ongoing measurement of key areas—such as customer service, automation, and breadth of supply chain line items—will serve as the justifying information needed for future strategic alignment. Additionally, using the same information-based approach in selecting optimal products for the organization will allow your organization's supply chain to manage only the items most needed, based on statistical and operational analyses.

Steps toward action:
1. Develop metrics around how products will be selected for your organization.
2. Define what key characteristics the partner vendor/manufacturer must have.
3. Communicate the vendor program mission and process to the key vendors/manufacturers for their understanding.
4. Receive leadership approval for process, content, and requirements.

Performance indicators/metrics:
- Cost reduction from item consolidation of high-cost and high-volume products
- Rate of compliance of vendor/manufacturers with newly implemented vendor program
- Compliance of clinical staff purchasing "optimal items" as determined by item analysis metrics

Project 6: Enhance Supply Chain Customer Communications

Supporting value principles:
- Be the master of the data.
- Increase staff knowledge of supply chain operations.

Financial impact estimate: Achieve a better working relationship and level of customer satisfaction through ongoing communication between clinical representatives and the supply chain. Financial impact will vary greatly by organization, so a conservative estimate is given.

Effort: Low
Benefit: Low

Cost estimates:
- Brainstorming session to launch new communication program (2–4 hours, including preparation time, for approximately $2,000)
- Supply chain operations staff member to manage periodic customer service meetings with clincial staff representatives, ensuring focus by product line (2 hours per week, for approximately $2,500 per year per organization)

Description: For this project, you will create a program of enhanced communciation between consuming customers (clinicians) and supporting supply chain areas, which will help with ongoing participation in supply chain initiatives. Communications will be kept productive and meaningful by using statistical information to facilitate communication about levels of documented customer service, product consolidation efforts, or item substitutions caused by outages, etc. Only by owning your own data can this platform of understanding be achieved and the clinical areas better understand the drivers and processes of supply chain operations. Clinical staff buy-in to supply chain efforts can be made more successful by establishing a platform of ongoing communications and by developing interpersonal relationships with supply chain team members.

Steps toward action:
1. Develop supply chain metrics.
2. Coordinate with departments to communicate desired project outcome and purpose.
3. Identify key participants in and schedule ongoing meetings.
4. Receive leadership approval for process, content, and requirements.
5. Evaluate metrics continuously.

Performance indicators/metrics:

- Clinical compliance with supply chain initiatives (minimization of resistance)
- Measures of supply chain customer service (proxy measured by number of item outages, response times, number of killed orders, etc.)

OTHER PROJECTS FOR CONSIDERATION

Project: Implement an Instrument Management System

Value principles: Clinical staff should focus on clinical decisions and patient care; develop supply chain goals and objectives by service line for medical/surgical items and pharmaceuticals.

Project: Develop a Contract Compliance Management Strategy

Value principle: Determine item, source, contract, and compliance targets for supply chain items of high cost and high volume.

Project: Develop the Clinically Efficient Supply Chain Model

Value principles: Clinical staff should focus on clinical decisions and patient care; and develop, standardize, and use supply chain metrics for quality, process, cost, and revenue production.

Project: Develop a Comprehensive Periodic Automatic Reordering Management Strategy

Value principles: Clinical staff should focus on clinical decisions and patient care; follow the supply items that bring in revenue; determine item, source, contract, and compliance targets for supply chain items of high cost and high volume; and develop, standardize, and use supply chain metrics for quality, process, cost, and revenue production.

Project: Implement Leading Practices and Operational Improvements to Affect Systemwide Local Inventory Reductions

Value principles: Develop, standardize, and use supply chain metrics for quality, process, cost, and revenue production; and develop supply chain goals and objectives by service line for medical/surgical items and pharmaceuticals.

Project: Create Centralized Oversight of Supply Chain Information Management

Value principle: Be the master of the data.

Project: Implement a Surgical Department/ Operating Room Perpetual Inventory

Value principles: Clinical staff should focus on clinical decisions and patient care; determine item, source, contract, and compliance targets for supply chain items of high cost and high volume; and develop supply chain goals and objectives by service line for medical/surgical items and pharmaceuticals.

SUMMARY

This chapter suggests various supply chain projects that are linked to value principles. Each project should be evaluated and adopted on its own merit, considering the specific situation of your healthcare organization. Projects can have incremental victories along the way to improving supply chain operations and management. The future of supply chain operations and management is discussed in summary fashion in the next chapter.

CHAPTER 5

Future Directions

The significant problems we face cannot be solved at the same level of thinking we were at when we created them.

—Albert Einstein

This book has discussed the importance of the strategic factors and value principles that can form the foundation of an effective healthcare supply chain system. Looking to the future, especially within the next ten years, the authors predict the occurrence of four important shifts in healthcare supply chain management: (1) organizational realignment; (2) integration of information systems and data; (3) merging of manufacturers, GPOs, distributors, and transportation organizations; and (4) the growth of customized pharmaceuticals and implants. ▶

ORGANIZATIONAL REALIGNMENT

A major realignment of healthcare supply chain management will occur at many locations, both at the hospital and at the healthcare system levels. Executive appointments with titles such as chief supply chain officer and vice president of supply chain will become more common. Cross-functional decision making will be guided through the establishment of "supply chain value analysis teams" (Burt 2006) and will include members that happen to be physicians, nurses, administrative officers, and other relevant stakeholders. Organizations will learn to appreciate that operational issues and even specific service-line supply item decisions are made more effectively in a collaborative and systematic fashion.

By outlining organizationwide supply chain goals and objectives and by making deliberate and open decisions on supply chain structures, a clear and concise direction can be shared by all internal stakeholders. It may prove advantageous for an organization to also include core external partners in discussions. Establishing organizationwide supply chain incentives can prove highly beneficial. Incentives can include bonuses and departmental rewards for success with supply chain goals. Medical staff incentives, to the extent permitted by law and deemed appropriate, should be considered. These incentives might include a percentage of savings going to medical research, the medical library, and so forth. Indeed, as a result of creative discussions by the team, all areas of the organization can earn rewards as a result of supply chain goal attainment.

A communications strategy that keeps the entire organization informed of supply chain challenges and strategies and the attainment of key goals is very important. Likewise, special steps need to be taken to ensure that members of governance (board members) are kept engaged in this whole process. Officers of the medical staff should also be conversant with the organization's supply chain mission, vision, and goals. Clinical and nonclinical employees should be kept informed of supply chain improvements, especially as appropriate for their area of work.

INTEGRATION OF INFORMATION SYSTEMS AND DATA

Total integration of information systems and data related to supply chain and other healthcare organization systems will allow for real success in the growing information-based healthcare culture. Utilizing electronic data interchange sets to replace current manual processes within the healthcare supply chain arena will permit easier and faster information sharing that is relevant to all stakeholders in the supply chain, from the manufacturer to the healthcare provider. Creating a method to periodically and thoroughly evaluate current IT functionality will allow for the ongoing adoption of updated software and technology appropriate for the organization.

Continuous development and training of staff on current and new applications and processes will allow for optimization of operational processes and of supply chain software being used. As industry pushes the integration efforts of healthcare information and supply chain data, it is critical that healthcare providers stay ahead of the imminent changes. Additionally, with greater need for disaster and terrorism readiness, having sound data upon which to make decisions is vital in the quest to remain appropriately prepared.

MERGING OF MANUFACTURERS, GPOS, DISTRIBUTORS, AND TRANSPORTATION ORGANIZATIONS

A growing trend toward the merging of manufacturers, GPOs, distributors, and transportation organizations is creating external semi–vertically integrated supply chain organizations that engage with healthcare providers and other markets. There is significant momentum in the effort to merge GPOs, distributors, transportation organizations, and in some cases manufacturers to provide a one-stop shop for health systems, hospitals, and other healthcare organizations. This will aid in aligning incentives, but clearly these will be externally motivated incentives. Healthcare providers must enter into these discussions to ensure better alignment of incentives, funding structures, process flows, and service and quality attributes that best meet healthcare provider and patient needs.

Merger activity will yield discussions involving everything from standardization of packaging strings and bar codes to the establishment of new delivery regions, routes, and frequencies. Healthcare providers have much to gain in joining in these discussions. Building external relationships, while having a firm foundation and solid understanding of one's own organizational needs, will help the organization systematically improve the healthcare supply chain across stakeholder groups.

CUSTOMIZED PHARMACEUTICALS AND IMPLANTS

There will be a continued push toward mass customization of key healthcare supply items. Paradoxically, there will be a concurrent, growing need for the ability to purchase highly differentiated items, especially customized pharmaceuticals and implants. These items will be as unique and specific as the genetic makeup of the end-using patient. This development will highlight the need for precision custom ordering and just-in-time delivery of customized supply items, and it will likewise require integrated information systems. The supply chain landscape will be greatly changed for healthcare organizations, especially as related to pharmaceuticals, orthopedics, and cardiac service lines.

Healthcare organizations that prepare for this shift away from current methods of distribution and toward shorter lead times and greater product specificity need to keep in mind the price of less-than-effective systems. Patients will certainly suffer if the genetically specific items are not there when needed. The supply chain system will also bear the brunt when these specific items are not available or when the wrong custom items are delivered. In these cases, the prospect of waste is great, because the custom items will likely be inappropriate for use by other patients. By necessity, information systems and methods of physical delivery will need to improve to accommodate the growth of custom patient implants and medications.

The healthcare supply chain will continue to be dynamic. Healthcare providers must work tirelessly toward building a more efficient and effective system that represents their own best interests, or they risk the reality that other stakeholders will lead the system to evolve according to their benefit. This would leave hospitals and health systems behind, and in more of a reactive mode, rather than in a proactive position. The bio-intelligence revolution has already begun; with it, there is a need for customized diagnostics, pharmaceuticals, and supplies. It is imperative that healthcare organizations restructure their supply chain while building external relationship bases. Regardless of the supply chain model (or hybrid model) adopted by a healthcare organization, the strategic factors and value principles presented in this book will prove to be the foundational and enabling tenets of a well-performing supply chain.

CONCLUSION

The two different supply chain models presented in this book, the traditional model and the vertically integrated model, represent two ends of the spectrum that will exist for healthcare providers into the future. Providers will need to make deliberate decisions as to which model to follow or what hybrid configuration will work best for them. In any event, the healthcare supply chain will evolve based on the forces of the marketplace. Healthcare organizations can affect that marketplace by understanding the models, by appreciating the trade-offs of outsourcing versus keeping components in-house, and by positively positioning the strategic factors that affect the supply chain. The supply chain value principles likewise are important to manage continuous incremental improvements in supply chain operations.

How the strategic factors and value principles fit within your organization should be the result of key leadership decisions, because they are powerful aids in the supply chain improvement process. Projects that are linked to value principles represent opportunities to jump-start the improvement process and to reinforce leadership commitment to optimizing the supply chain.

Healthcare leadership therefore must accept the challenge to shape the future. This can be done by better aligning incentives with needs, by developing and continuously improving supply chain processes, by integrating with other vital elements of the business of care delivery, and by bolstering the supply chain operational competence of all team members. The rewards for attending to strategic factors and value principles, as discussed in this book, can be great for the healthcare organization. Following this process can provide an organizational foundation that is solid and endures into a dynamic future. Following this process can yield significant improvements to physician, nurse, and staff satisfaction; to the financial bottom line; and, most importantly, to patient safety and quality patient care.

REFERENCE

Burt, T. 2006. "Seeing the Future: Innovative Supply Chain Management Strategies." *Healthcare Executive* 21 (1): 16–21.

ABOUT THE AUTHORS

GERALD R. LEDLOW, PH.D., M.H.A, FACHE. Dr. Ledlow is graduate program director in health services policy and management at the Jiann-Ping Hsu College of Public Health at Georgia Southern University in Statesboro. Previously, Dr. Ledlow was the corporate vice president for supply chain at the Genesis Project, a Sisters of Mercy Health System initiative to redesign the delivery of healthcare services, specifically focusing on supply chain processes. Dr. Ledlow is a Fellow of the American College of Healthcare Executives and has more than 20 years of healthcare experience in supply chain, logistics, facility management, and managed care. Dr. Ledlow earned his doctorate degree in organizational leadership from the University of Oklahoma in Norman; master's degree in healthcare administration from Baylor University in Waco, Texas; and bachelor's degree in economics from the Virginia Military Institute in Lexington. He has been a coauthor of and contributor to many publications and is a national and international speaker on various topics in healthcare. Dr. Ledlow can be reached at gledlow@ georgiasouthern.edu.

ALLISON P. CORRY, M.H.A, M.B.A. Ms. Corry is a senior consultant for ARAMARK Healthcare–Supply Chain Management Services. Previously, she was a senior consultant for the Genesis Project. Ms. Corry is an active member of the American College of Healthcare Executives. She earned her master's degrees in healthcare administration and in business administration as well as her bachelor of science degree from the University of Missouri in Columbia. Her primary academic foci were in the areas of healthcare supply chain and operational logistics. Ms. Corry can be reached at corry-allison@aramark.com.

MARK A. CWIEK, J.D., M.H.A, FACHE. Dr. Cwiek is the director of the health administration division of the Central Michigan University School of Health Sciences in Mount Pleasant. He has more than a decade of service as a faculty member at Central Michigan University and is a tenured professor. Dr. Cwiek also has more than 15 years of experience as in-house legal counsel, hospital executive, and chief executive officer of hospitals and healthcare systems. He is widely published and is a Fellow of the American College of Healthcare Executives. Dr. Cwiek received his juris doctorate degree and master degree in healthcare administration from St. Louis University in Missouri and his bachelor of science degree in psychology and German from Wayne State University in Detroit, Michigan. He can be reached at cwiek1ma@cmich.edu.